EMERGENCY MEDICINE:

AN INTRODUCTORY GUIDE

NEIL PATEL, M.D.
ASSISTANT CLINICAL PROFESSOR OF MEDICINE
DAVID GEFFEN SCHOOL OF MEDICINE AT UCLA
ATTENDING PHYSICIAN
DIVISION OF EMERGENCY MEDICINE
WEST LOS ANGELES VA MEDICAL CENTER

Copyright 2014
Rev: 8.3.2014

TABLE OF CONTENTS

INTRODUCTION

While rotating through the emergency department, you will gain experience addressing a diverse range of clinical presentations. Unlike other fields of medicine, there is not a limitation based on organ system, age, gender, etc. with respect to who is able to come into the Emergency Department. As such, you must rely upon a vast range of knowledge in order to successfully care for emergency department patients.

While this can seem somewhat overwhelming, it is important to remember that our principal role is to evaluate patients for possible *life- or limb-threatening causes* of their chief complaint and not necessarily to come to a firm conclusion about the underlying etiology of their symptoms. For instance, if a patient is experiencing chest pain, the emergency physician will want to ensure that all life-threating causes (acute coronary syndrome, pulmonary embolism, aortic dissection, mediastinitis, etc.) have been ruled-out before discharging the patient home with a defined plan for further outpatient care where the ultimate non-urgent cause of their chest pain may be elucidated and treated (i.e. costochondritis, muscular strain/sprain).

As you can see, emergency medicine employs a *deductive reasoning* approach to evaluating patients rather than the *inductive reasoning* paradigm with which you may be more familiar. Deductive reasoning relies on *ruling-out* disease processes whereas an inductive approach is used to *rule-in* diseases. In other words, while fields such as internal medicine are geared towards discovery of the exact, ultimate cause of the patient's symptoms, emergency medicine is focused upon trying to exclude life-threating diseases processes. Therefore, during your work in the emergency department, it will be essential for you to know and understand what these potential life- and limb-threatening disease processes are for varied patient complaints.

With this goal in mind, each of the following chapters focuses on a different chief complaint commonly encountered in the emergency department. Within each chapter, I present 5 to 10 dangerous, life-threatening disease processes that must be entertained as part of the "dangerous differential" for each chief complaint. We will review the common historical features and physical exam findings that typically characterize each of these disease processes. In certain cases, we will also review the work-up and treatment options available for some of these disease processes. While I will focus on the most typical, "textbook" presentations of these diseases, it is very important to realize that the same disease can present in many different ways and that not all patients will experience all of the signs and symptoms which you might typically expect. While at times frustrating, this is what makes our work exciting and challenging and this is where having experience matters, so please try to see as many patients as safely possible!

It is my sincere hope that these pages will not only help you gain a better appreciation of emergency medicine and expand your knowledge base, but most importantly, will help you in providing excellent, thoughtful care for all your future patients.

CHAPTER 1: CHEST PAIN

Chest pain is one of the most frequent complaints encountered in the Emergency Department, especially at the West LA VA Medical Center. There are literally hundreds of pathologies – both life-threating and benign – that could result in a patient experiencing pain in their anterior thorax. Having to discover the cause of everyone's chest pain would be a Herculean task. Fortunately, as providers of emergency care, it is our responsibility to specifically evaluate for life- or limb-threatening causes of a patient's chest pain. While the differential that we must consider is more constrained, it is nonetheless fraught with peril in that atypical presentations are common and morbidity and mortality may ensure if the diagnosis is not made in a timely fashion.

The "dangerous differential" for chest pain includes:

- Acute coronary syndrome (includes unstable angina, NSTEMI and STEMI)
- Pulmonary embolism
- Aortic dissection
- Pneumothorax
- Pericarditis
- Pneumonia
- Esophageal rupture (Borhaave's syndrome)
- Pleural effusion

ACUTE CORONARY SYNDROME

HISTORY: The classic description of anginal chest pain includes a substernal pressure-like sensation or tightness with radiation down the left arm, neck or jaw (though radiation down the right arm has been shown to be more specific for ACS!), associated with shortness of breath, nausea and diaphoresis. However, it is important to remember that this classic description doesn't hold true for all patients. In particular, women, the elderly and diabetic patients often have atypical presentations that may be difficult to localize due to the visceral nature of the symptoms experienced during coronary vascular occlusion. Some patients may not experience outright discomfort, but may instead report symptoms resulting from a decreased cardiac output (lightheadedness, dyspnea). Therefore, one must carefully ascertain the history, making sure to pay attention to details of time of onset, provoking and palliating features and background risk factors for coronary artery disease.

PHYSICAL EXAM: The physical exam of a patient experiencing ACS may be rather benign though a patient experiencing active coronary occlusion may appear to be pale, diaphoretic and in marked respiratory distress. The physical exam should be used predominantly to exclude other causes of chest pain (zoster, pneumothorax, pleural effusion, pneumonia, etc.) One important point to note is that reproducible chest pain does NOT rule-out acute coronary syndrome. In fact, approximately 15% of patients with ACS will have a reproducible component of their chest pain.

WORK-UP: The work-up for ACS relies predominately on the history, ECG and cardiac biomarkers. Once these elements have been obtained, the patient is placed in a risk-category (low, medium or high) based upon the AHA/ACC 2008 ACS guidelines. Once an MI has been ruled-out (negative cardiac biomarkers 12 hours after the onset of the patient's last chest pain), low-risk patients can be discharged home with a follow-up appointment for a risk stratification study (exercise treadmill test, nuclear myocardial perfusion imaging, stress echocardiography, etc.) within 72 hours. Intermediate risk patients can either be admitted to the Telemetry service for further inpatient risk stratification or be placed in "cardiac observation" in which the patient will get serial ECGs and cardiac biomarkers (to rule-out MI) and undergo a formal cardiology evaluation to determine the best course of action. Patients meeting any of the high-risk criteria should be admitted to the Telemetry service for further inpatient risk stratification and possible cardiac catheterization.

TREATMENT: Treatment for ACS from the emergency department focuses on providing the patient with agents that inhibit primary and secondary hemostasis. Primary hemostasis involves platelet function and should be inhibited with aspirin (minimum dose 162mg chewed). Other anti-platelet agents such as clopidogrel and the GpIIbIIIa inhibitors will usually be given by the cardiology service. The secondary hemostasis pathway involves the clotting cascade and is inhibited with agents such as heparin and enoxaparin. These agents are typically reserved for high-risk ACS patients. Nitroglycerin should be given to increase myocardial oxygen supply via dilation of coronary arteries.

In patients with an acute ST-elevation MI (STEMI), the priority is on achieving timely reperfusion of the obstructed coronary vessel. Reperfusion may be achieved via activation of tertiary hemostasis (activation of tissue plasminogen) by using TPA or via direct coronary catheterization and deployment of a stent across the stenotic vessel. These patients should receive aspirin, clopidogrel and heparin before going to the catheterization lab or receiving TPA.

PULMONARY EMBOLISM

HISTORY: Patients with pulmonary embolism will classically report an acute, sharp, pleuritic chest pain without radiation associated with shortness of breath. If the source of the pulmonary embolus is a lower extremity deep venous thrombosis (DVT), the patient may report asymmetric lower extremity edema/swelling. The pain typically does not radiate. The patient may relate a history of recent immobilization or may have an underlying malignancy.

PHYSICAL EXAMINATION: Patients with PE typically will have resting tachycardia, varying degrees of hypoxia and possible tachypnea. The patient may also exhibit hemoptysis. In patients with a massive PE, hypotension may also be noted. It is important to note that these findings are not necessarily present in all patients with pulmonary embolism and many patients with PE may demonstrate relatively normal vital signs.

WORK-UP: The work-up of PE relies on the establishment of a pre-test probability of having a PE. Using the Wells Criteria, if a patient is low-risk for PE, a d-dimer may be ordered and if high, a CT Pulmonary Angiogram or a V/Q scan can be ordered to evaluate for the presence of PE. If the Wells Criteria reveal the patient to be intermediate or high-risk, the patient should undergo radiographic testing directly.

TREATMENT: The treatment of most pulmonary emboli relies of preventing the development of further thrombus by administering heparin. If the patient is in obstructive shock (hypotensive, severely tachycardic), there is limited evidence for the use of thrombolytics in this clinical setting. Patients with PE should be admitted to a monitored setting.

AORTIC DISSECTION

HISTORY: Patients with aortic dissection classically will describe an acute onset, sharp, severe tearing anterior chest pain that radiates to the back. Patients can demonstrate features of Marfan's syndrome (lanky, thin, elongated digits), which is a risk factor for aortic dissection. It is very important to note that the above classic description doesn't apply to the majority of patients with aortic dissection. Instead, rely upon a history of an acute-onset, severe chest pain to entertain the diagnosis of aortic dissection.

PHYSICAL EXAM: Many textbooks mention a difference in blood pressure between both arms in patients with aortic dissection. However, this has been shown to only be 15% sensitive and is not specific for aortic dissection. Most patients with aortic dissection will be hypertensive and a palpable pulse deficit has been shown to be more sensitive than a blood pressure difference in detecting aortic dissection.

WORK-UP: Aortic dissection is commonly diagnosed via a CT Angiogram of the chest and abdomen. Alternative imaging strategies involve a transesophageal echocardiogram or a magnetic resonance (MR) angiogram.

TREATMENT: In patients with type A dissections (involving any part of the aorta proximal to the ligamentum arteriosum), surgical and medical interventions are indicated. In type B dissections (involving only that part of the aorta distal to the ligamentum arteriosum), a medical approach is undertaken. The medical treatment of aortic dissection involves first giving an agent to decrease the heart rate and then giving an agent to reduce blood pressure so as to decrease the shear stress on the aortic wall.

PNEUMOTHORAX

HISTORY: Patients with a pneumothorax will often describe an acute onset, mild/moderate sharp, pleuritic chest pain associated with shortness of breath. Patients with a primary spontaneous pneumothorax will often be tall and thin whereas patients with a secondary spontaneous pneumothorax will have underlying pulmonary disease such as COPD.

PHYSICAL EXAM: Patients with a pneumothorax will often exhibit absent breath sounds over the area of the pneumothorax. In addition, they may exhibit increased tympani to percussion over the area of the pneumothorax.

PERICARDITIS

HISTORY: Patients with pericarditis may report a sharp pleuritic chest pain that classically is worse with lying flat and better with leaning forward. There is often a history of a recent viral infection.

PHYSICAL EXAMINATION: Patients with pericarditis may exhibit a pericardial friction rub, though this is rather difficult to appreciate, especially in a loud and busy emergency department. If there is an associated large pericardial effusion, the patient may exhibit tachycardia, hypotension, distended JVP and muffled heart sounds (Beck's triad).

CHAPTER 2: SHORTNESS OF BREATH

You will encounter many patients whose chief complaint is dyspnea or shortness of breath. While at times the disease process is rather obvious, such as when a patient with asthma presents with an acute exacerbation, in other instances the underlying diagnosis may require a much more considered approach. Given that breathing is such a critical function of life, the symptom of not being able to breath normally more likely than not portends a significant underlying pathologic process that we must rapidly ascertain and promptly begin to treat. The "dangerous differential" for shortness of breath or dyspnea includes:

- Pulmonary edema
- Obstructive airway diseases (includes asthma and COPD)
- Pleural effusion
- Pneumonia
- Pulmonary embolism
- Restrictive airway diseases (includes pulmonary fibrosis)
- Pneumothorax
- Acute coronary syndrome
- Anemia

PULMONARY EDEMA

HISTORY: Patients may develop pulmonary edema from several different sources. Most commonly, you will encounter the patient with congestive heart failure. Patients with an acute CHF exacerbation will likely report dyspnea that is worse with exertion and with lying down in a recumbent position. In addition, if there is concomitant right-sided heart failure, the patient may report weight gain and edema in dependent portions of the body (lower extremities, scrotum, etc.).

PHYSICIAL EXAM: The physical exam of a patient with CHF will likely reveal inspiratory crackles upon pulmonary auscultation as well as a distended JVP, bilateral lower extremity pitting edema and an S3 heart sound may be appreciated resulting from blood rushing into a dilated ventricle during diastole. The crackles appreciated on pulmonary auscultation of a patient with pulmonary edema result from alveoli, which are filled with fluid, "popping" open during inspiration.

WORK-UP: The work-up of a patient with pulmonary edema resulting from CHF relies upon determining why an exacerbation occurred in the first place since the diagnosis is often made upon clinical grounds. A history of medication or dietary non-compliance may explain an exacerbation or possible cardiac ischemia/infarction may have further reduced the ejection fraction and thereby the cardiac output of the patient. A BNP may be of limited help in those patients in whom the diagnosis of pulmonary edema is not obvious, though a chest x-ray often can also lend corroborating evidence.

TREATMENT: The treatment of an acute CHF exacerbation relies upon three main principles: 1) reduction of preload to lower LVEDV such that a higher cardiac output can result according to the Frank-Starling principle; 2) reduction of afterload to reduce the workload on the ventricle; and 3) increasing cardiac contractility to promote an increase in cardiac output and resultant organ perfusion. Preload and afterload can both be rapidly reduced via the use of nitroglycerin. Furosemide also reduces preload but may take hours to be effective, whereas nitrates work much more immediately. IV ACE-inhibitors can also be used to rapidly reduce preload without compromising cardiac contractility as would occur if beta-blockers were to be used. It is indeed an important concept to remember that negative ionotropic agents such as beta-blockers should NOT be used in an acute CHF exacerbation, despite the long-term benefits that they have been shown to have upon cardiac remodeling when used in patients with stable, well-controlled CHF.

OBSTRUCTIVE AIRWAY DISEASES

HISTORY: Patients with asthma and COPD will often report wheezing and may endorse a cough or a recent history of a viral URI. They may relate a history of exposure to environmental agents which may have precipitated their exacerbation, but this is not necessary. Most patients whom you encounter in the emergency department will likely have an established history or asthma or COPD so it is important to ask patients about their relevant past pulmonary history.

PHYSICAL EXAM: The physical exam of a patient with a asthma or COPD exacerbation will likely reveal expiratory and/or inspiratory wheezing, accessory muscle use, a prolonged expiratory phase (hence "obstructive" airway disease), and tachypnea with an increased work of breathing.

WORK-UP: The work-up of patients with COPD or asthma exacerbations in the emergency department centers around ascertaining the underlying reason for the exacerbation and ruling-out any associated complications such as a pneumothorax or lobar collapse. A CXR is usually helpful in terms of ruling-out pneumonia as well as possible other causes of the patient's wheezing such as pulmonary edema.

TREATMENT: Treatment of asthma and COPD is in general rather similar. The treatment strategy for both involves administering β_2-agonists and anti-cholinergic agents via nebulization. In addition, the inflammatory process contributing to the exacerbation is ameliorated via the administration of steroids such as prednisone or dexamethasone.

Antibiotics are reserved for those patients with COPD with a change in the character of their sputum or in asthmatics with a proven pneumonia.

PLEURAL EFFUSION

Patients may develop a pleural effusion from varied sources. Transudative effusions usually result from increased venous hydrostatic pressure (CHF) or a low oncotic pressure state (hepatic cirrhosis, nephrotic syndrome). Exudative effusions usually are infectious in nature and result as a complication of a severe pneumonia.

HISTORY: Patients with a pleural effusion will report dyspnea that is often improved by lying on one side or another. In addition, they may report a dull "ache" in their chest or back. There will usually be a history of an underlying disease process contributing to the effusion (malignancy, cirrhosis, CHF) as pleural effusions rarely develop spontaneously in the absence of other pathologies.

PHYSICAL EXAM: The physical exam of a patient with a pleural effusion will reveal decreased breath sounds over the area of the effusion. In addition, there will be a *decrease* in tactile fremitus as there is now fluid interposed between the lung and the parietal pleura. The presence of egophany (when the patients says "E", upon auscultation it sounds like the patient is instead saying "A") may also be noted. Moreover, one may appreciate bronchial breath sounds if the pressure exerted from the pleural effusion collapses the aleveolar sacs surrounding a respiratory bronchus.

WORK-UP: A pleural effusion can be appreciated on physical exam. Chest radiography and less often, ultrasound are the mainstays of making this diagnosis in the emergency department. Once an effusion is found, the source of the effusion must be identified. Use of Light's Criteria will help in classifying the effusion as either transudative or exudative.

TREATMENT: While the ultimate treatment of a pleural effusion depends upon its underlying etiology, an effusion causing significant respiratory distress should be drained via thoracentesis in the emergency department.

PNEUMONIA

HISTORY: Patients with pneumonia will often report a history of fever and a productive cough. Classic, typical pneumonias (usually associated with *S. pneumoniae* and *S. aureus*) will present with an acute onset high fever. In contrast, atypical pneumonias (traditionally associated with mycoplasma, legionella, etc.) may present only with low-grade temperatures and several days of indolent symptoms with a typically non-productive cough.

PHYSICAL EXAM: The physical exam of a patient with pneumonia may reveal inspiratory crackles which represent alveoli filled with pus that "pop" open upon adequate inspiration in that area of the lung affected by the pneumonia. A pleural effusion may also be appreciated in some patients with pneumonia (a para-pneumonic effusion). This para-pneumonic effusion may later organize into an abscess which will need to be drained (either by chest tube or pigtail catheter insertion) in order to achieve adequate resolution.

WORK-UP: Pneumonia is traditionally diagnosed on the basis of the history, exam and chest radiography. Indeed, the IDSA 2007 pneumonia treatment guidelines stipulate that there must be x-ray evidence of a pneumonia in order for this diagnosis to be made.

TREATMENT: Depending upon the patient's co-morbidities and specific risk factors (i.e. recent hospitalization, nursing home or dialysis patient), particular antibiotics or combinations of antibiotics are administered. Good pulmonary toilet techniques (deep inspiration, chest percussion) are also important – though often overlooked – elements in the treatment of pneumonia.

CHAPTER 3: UPPER ABDOMINAL PAIN

Abdominal pain is one of the most frequent complaints among patients who visit the emergency department. The abdominal and pelvic cavities contain many structures which can experience a myriad of acute-life threatening pathologies. This fact combined with the visceral, amorphous nature of the pain relayed by these structures makes the diagnosis of critical intraabdominal pathologies particularly challenging. Since there are so many complex diagnoses related to the abdomen, for convenience, I have divided our consideration into pathologies involving the upper abdomen with those diseases presenting as pain in the lower abdomen to be discussed in the following section.

When considering pain in the upper abdomen, whether right, left or epigastric, it is best to take an anatomical approach with consideration of each of the structures within and adjacent to the area where pain is being experienced. For instance, when considering pain in the left upper quadrant, one must consider not only pathologies involving the stomach, spleen, lower esophagus and colon, but diseases of the heart, lower lungs and kidney should also be entertained as pain resulting from pathologies in these structures is visceral in nature with poor somatic localization. With this in mind, the "dangerous differential" of pain in the upper abdomen includes:

- Acute cholecystitis
- Acute ascending cholangitis
- Acute hepatitis
- Acute pancreatitis
- Ruptured gastric or duodenal ulcer
- Mesenteric ischemia
- Acute coronary syndrome
- Pneumonia

ACUTE CHOLECYSTITIS

Acute cholecystitis results from obstruction of the cystic duct (usually by an impacted gallstone) which then leads to venous congestion of the gallbladder wall. This venous congestion then impedes arterial inflow allowing necrosis and invasion of the gallbladder wall by bacterial pathogens. This process sets up a possibly life-threatening process that can lead to death via overwhelming sepsis.

HISTORY: Patients with acute cholecystitis usually have a preceding history of months to years of colicky post-prandial RUQ or epigastric abdominal pain, especially after eating foods high in fat (fatty acids stimulate the release of cholecystokinin which causes gallbladder wall contraction). When these patients are in the throes of acute cholecystitis, they may present with a fever and prolonged, constant RUQ pain as opposed to short bouts of colicky RUQ pain experienced with symptomatic cholelithiasis.

PHYSICAL EXAM: The physical exam will often reveal inspiratory arrest upon deep palpation of the RUQ (a positive Murphy's sign) along with the possible presence of a fever. The patient typically will NOT be jaundiced with acute cholecystitis since the hepatic ducts and common bile duct are usually patent and excess bile can still be drained into the duodenum.

WORK-UP: The diagnosis of acute cholecystitis is principally made using ultrasound in which gallbladder wall thickening and pericholecystic fluid can be seen. A nuclear medicine test known as a HIDA scan can also be used to look for obstruction of the cystic duct indicating likely cholecystitis.

TREATMENT: Treatment of acute cholecystitis is with a combination of antibiotics and surgical cholecystectomy. Antibiotics should cover enterobacteriaceae as well as anaerobes. Ceftriaxone and metronidazole in combination should suffice for most cases.

ACUTE ASCENDING CHOLANGITIS

Acute ascending cholangitis results from an obstruction of the common bile duct (again most commonly from a gallstone) with resultant infection and inflammation of the biliary ducts.

HISTORY: Patients with acute ascending cholangitis will typically report a fever as well as a constant RUQ abdominal pain. Family members may relate a history of new onset jaundice. Indeed, the combination of fever, jaundice and right upper quadrant abdominal pain forms Charcot's triad, which describes the classic findings with acute ascending cholangitis.

PHYSICAL EXAM: The physical exam will likely reveal the presence of a fever, tenderness in the right upper quadrant as well as jaundice. Patient with acute ascending cholangitis tend to be rather ill-appearing and may meet criteria for sepsis.

WORK-UP: The diagnosis of acute ascending cholangitis is classically clinical, but ultrasound can help detect the presence of a dilated common bile duct.

TREATMENT: The treatment of acute ascending cholangitis involves a combination of broad-spectrum antibiotics (covering anaerobes and enterobacteriaceae), early goal-directed therapy for sepsis (if present), and emergent endoscopic retrograde cholangiopacreatography (ERCP) to remove the offending obstructing stone from the common bile duct. These patients are typically admitted to an ICU setting.

ACUTE HEPATITIS

HISTORY: Acute hepatitis can occur from infectious, chemical or ischemic sources. However, most acute forms of severe hepatitis that we encounter in the emergency department will be from an infectious etiology (Hepatitis A, E, EBV, etc.). Patients may relay a history of a viral prodrome or recent travel (in the case of Hepatitis A and E). Family members may note the presence of jaundice in the patient and if severe, may also report that the patient is confused from baseline.

PHYSICAL EXAM: The physical exam of a patient with acute hepatitis will likely reveal a tender, enlarged liver in the presence of clinical jaundice.

WORK-UP: Acute hepatitis is often diagnosed on the basis of jaundice and the presence of elevated hepatic enzymes (AST/ALT). Titers for Hepatitis A through E, EBV, etc. can be sent to determine if a particular viral agent is responsible.

TREATMENT: Treatment for acute hepatitis is largely supportive. In cases of acute fulminant hepatic failure, allogeneic liver transplantation may be considered.

ACUTE PANCREATITIS

HISTORY: Patients with acute pancreatitis often describe severe epigastric pain that radiates to the back (likely because the pancreas is a retroperitoneal structure) associated with intense nausea/vomiting and anorexia.

PHYSICAL EXAM: Patients with acute pancreatitis often appear to be in acute distress and may exhibit significant epigastric tenderness to palpation. In addition, if the patient has acute necrotizing pancreatitis, s/he may exhibit a fever as well as signs or symptoms of sepsis. Moreover, patients with acute hemorrhagic pancreatitis may exhibit ecchymosis along either flank (from blood collected in the retroperitoneum) known as the Grey-Turner sign.

WORK-UP: Besides the above clinical clues, an elevated lipase is both sensitive and specific for acute pancreatitis. Amylase was the former test of choice for the diagnosis of acute pancreatitis, but owing to poor specificity and equal sensitivity to lipase, is no longer routinely used for this diagnosis. CT imaging with intravenous contrast can sometimes help discern if the patient is having acute necrotizing or hemorrhagic pancreatitis.

14

TREATMENT: The mainstay of treatment for acute pancreatitis is to make the patient NPO (so as to prevent the release of further lipase from the injured pancreas), IV fluids and pain medications. In patients with acute necrotizing pancreatitis, broad-spectrum antibiotics such as meropenem are added.

RUPTURED GASTRIC OR DUODENAL ULCER

HISTORY: Patients with a ruptured ulcer will often be able to relate the exact time of pain onset. The pain tends to be extremely intense and since there is rupture of a hollow viscus, gastric and duodenal contents will spill into the peritoneal cavity causing peritonitis and a much more generalized abdominal pain. Patients may have a pre-existing history of peptic ulcer disease.

PHYSICAL EXAM: In patients with a ruptured ulcer, the abdomen tends to be diffusely tender and rigid with peritoneal signs (rebound tenderness and involuntary guarding). As time progresses, these patients will gradually decompensate and appear to be quite ill. This is one of the limited range of pathologies that will lead to the presence of a true "surgical abdomen" on physical exam (diffuse involuntary guarding and rebound tenderness).

WORK-UP: The diagnosis is often made on clinical grounds, but a CT scan may reveal the source of perforation as well as free air in the peritoneal cavity.

TREATMENT: The treatment for a ruptured ulcer is emergent exploratory laparotomy to first discover the source of perforation and then to repair the defect in the bowel wall. The patient should promptly be started on a proton-pump inhibitor drip to deactivate pepsin so as to prevent it from digesting intraperitoneal structures.

ACUTE MESENTERIC ISCHEMIA

Acute mesenteric ischemia results from a lack of oxygenation of the small and/or large intestine, eventually leading to necrosis, compromise of bowel-wall integrity and spillage of intestinal contents within the peritoneal cavity. It is generally thought to be due to one of four processes: 1) acute embolus to one of the mesenteric vessels, 2) thrombotic occlusion of one of the mesenteric vessels, 3) vasoconstriction of the mesenteric vessels (such as from being on a norepinephrine drip or using cocaine), or 4) having a thrombus within one of the mesenteric veins.

HISTORY: Patients with acute mesenteric ischemia, especially the embolic subtype (most common) will often report an acute onset of progressively severe abdominal pain. These patients will often have a source for the embolism and therefore may carry a diagnosis such as atrial fibrillation. Patients with the thrombotic subtype will often report a history of progressively worsening post-prandial abdominal pain and may even report phagophobia (a fear of eating) as it often results in pain for the patient. Patients with this subtype may also exhibit many of the classic cardiovascular risk factors such as diabetes, hypertension, hyperlipidemia and tobacco use. Patients with the non-occlusive subtype will either be on an agent that decreases splanchnic blood flow (e.g. norepinephrine, octreotide) or may report a history of cocaine use. Patients with a mesenteric venous thrombus will typically have a history of a previous DVT/PE or may report a family history of a prothrombotic state such as Factor V Leiden, Protein C or S deficiency, or Prothrombin G20210A mutation. In either case, in the acute setting of vascular compromise, these patients will all report a severe, oftentimes vague, diffuse abdominal pain that progressively worsens.

PHYSICAL EXAM: The physical exam of a patient with mesenteric ischemia classically will reveal pain out of proportion to exam. This is to say that despite the lack of hard physical findings such as guarding and rebound tenderness, the patient exhibits pain that is out of proportion with a seemingly benign abdominal exam. Later in the course, as intestinal ischemia and eventually perforation set in, the patient may exhibit true peritoneal signs of involuntary guarding and rebound tenderness.

WORK-UP: Mesenteric ischemia is oftentimes a difficult diagnosis to make. One must rely upon the presence of relevant risk factors in the setting of a history of acute onset, progressively worsening abdominal pain. CT of the abdomen and pelvis may reveal thickening of the bowel in the distribution of the involved vasculature and rarely, a filling defect in the involved vessel can be appreciated if the contrast bolus is administered at the correct time. Contrary to popular belief, there is no commonly used laboratory test (e.g. lactate and LDH) that is sensitive or specific for the diagnosis of mesenteric ischemia.

TREATMENT: The treatment of mesenteric ischemia requires prompt revasularization and resection of any necrotic bowel. Therefore, interventional radiology (IR) may be consulted to perform an angiogram with injection of papaverine to digest the offending clot. Surgery should additionally be consulted so that necrotic bowel can be excised before frank perforation occurs.

CHAPTER 4: LOWER ABDOMINAL PAIN

Just as with upper abdominal pain, there are a myriad of pathologies that may present as pain in the lower abdomen. Again, owing to the visceral nature of many of these diseases, the area of perceived pain may not necessarily correspond to the anatomical location of the structure responsible. For instance, diseases involving the genital organs often present as pain in the lower abdomen rather than as pain in the scrotum or pelvis. With this is mind, the "dangerous differential" for pain in the lower abdomen includes:

- Acute appendicitis
- Acute diverticulitis
- Acute volvulus
- Acute cystitis
- Testicular/Ovarian torsion
- Epididymo-orchitis
- Pelvic inflammatory disease (PID)

ACUTE APPENDICITIS

HISTORY: Patients with acute appendicitis will traditionally report the gradual onset of a diffuse periumbilical abdominal pain which later localizes to the right lower quadrant. Patients will also often experience anorexia, nausea/vomiting and fever. However, as appendicitis is a very common disease process, atypical presentations will be seen with some regularity.

PHYSICAL EXAM: By surface anatomy, the appendix is classically located at a point two-thirds of the way between the umbilicus and the right anterior superior iliac spine (McBurney's point). When the parietal peritoneum is brought in contact with the inflamed appendix at this point by manual palpation, the pain experienced by the adjacent parietal peritoneum will result in significant tenderness and guarding. Indeed, tenderness at the right lower quadrant is one of the most specific tests for acute appendicitis. Patients may also exhibit a positive psoas sign (pain with flexion of the right hip), obturator sign (pain with internal and external rotation of the right hip) and Rovsing's sign (pain in the right lower quadrant elicited by palpation of the left lower quadrant).

WORK-UP: The diagnosis of acute appendicitis is mostly made on clinical grounds. However, CT of the abdomen and pelvis is being used with increasing frequency to make this diagnosis, ostensibly to decrease the rate of negative laparotomies. In pregnant women and children, ultrasound can be used to diagnose appendicitis. However, it is important to remember that ultrasound, while specific for appendicitis, is not at all very sensitive for this diagnosis. Therefore, in the setting of a negative or indeterminate ultrasound result, one must pursue further imaging with a CT abdomen/pelvis.

TREATMENT: The treatment of acute appendicitis remains surgical excision. In the setting of perforated appendicitis, the patient may be admitted for several days of IV antibiotics with delayed surgical appendectomy. IV antibiotics covering enteric flora (enterobacteriaceae and anaerobes) should be given, though evidence for this is somewhat limited.

ACUTE DIVERTICULITIS

HISTORY: Patients with acute diverticulitis may report a gradual onset of progressively worsening pain, usually in the left lower quadrant as most cases of diverticulitis occur in the sigmoid colon from an obstruction and consequent infection of a pre-existing diverticulum.

PHYSICAL EXAM: The physical exam of a patient with acute diverticulitis often reveals tenderness to palpation with or without guarding in the left lower quadrant of the abdomen.

WORK-UP: The diagnosis is often made by CT of the abdomen/pelvis, though in patients having recurrent flares who are otherwise well-appearing without peritoneal signs (indicating perforation), the diagnosis may be made clinically and treatment started on a presumptive basis.

TREATMENT: The treatment for acute diverticulitis is largely medical with antibiotics covering enteric flora (enterobacteriaceae and anaerobes). In patients with more than two flares, referral to a colorectal surgeon for consideration of a sigmoidectomy should be made. Patients with an acute flare of diverticulitis should NOT undergo a colonoscopy for fear of causing a perforation.

ACUTE VOLVULUS

HISTORY: Patients who experience an acute sigmoid volvulus tend to be elderly and oftentimes bedbound. They may report an acute onset of left lower quadrant or a more diffuse abdominal pain, possibly associated with vomiting and obstipation (failure to pass gas or stool).

PHYSICAL EXAM: The physical exam of a patient with volvulus may reveal an area of increased tympani in the abdomen along with tenderness on the left side of the abdomen.

WORK-UP: Sigmoid volvulus can be diagnosed by plain radiography or more commonly, with CT of the abdomen/pelvis.

TREATMENT: Sigmoidoscopy can be performed in cases of sigmoid volvulus in an attempt to untwist the involved bowel. However, surgery remains the definitive treatment of choice.

ACUTE CYSTITIS

HISTORY: Patient with acute cystitis will usually report a history of dysuria, urgency and frequency. Men with cystitis usually have a predisposing condition such as benign prostatic hyperplasia (BPH) with urinary retention.

PHYSICAL EXAM: Patients with cystitis may exhibit tenderness in the suprapubic region overlying the bladder.

WORK-UP: Cystitis can be diagnosed on the basis of a routine urine analysis.

TREATMENT: Treatment is with antibiotics, typically covering *E. coli* and other gram-negative rods.

TESTICULAR/OVARIAN TORSION

HISTORY: Patients with gonadal torsion will often report a history of unilateral acute-onset, intermittent pain in either the scrotum or lower abdomen/pelvis associated with nausea and possibly vomiting. These episodes may last minutes to a few hours representing torsion and spontaneous detorsion.

PHYSICAL EXAM: In cases of testicular torsion, one may note that the involved testis lies in an abnormal, oftentimes horizontal plane and is sometimes edematous and tender to palpation owing to ischemia and venous congestion. Classically, there is a lack of a cremasteric reflex and failure of pain to improve with elevation of the testis (negative Prehn's sign). However, this latter test (Prehn's test) has been shown to be rather unreliable in differentiating testicular torsion from epididymo-orchitis.

The physical exam of ovarian torsion may reveal a fullness in the involved adenexa representing a possible ovarian cyst or other lead point around which the torsion occurred (i.e. around which the vascular pedicle twisted).

WORK-UP: Since time is of the essence, torsion should be diagnosed based on clinical grounds and the relevant consultants immediately called since timely surgical detorsion and fixation are necessary to preserve gonadal function. However, owing to diagnostic uncertainty in many cases, ultrasound is often used to evaluate for blood flow to the involved gonad. However, it is important to remember that in cases when spontaneous detorsion has occurred the vascular supply by Doppler ultrasound will appear to be intact. Therefore, if the diagnosis is still suspected based on clinical grounds, the relevant consultant must still be involved in the care of the patient.

TREATMENT: As stated above, timely (preferably within 6 hours) surgical detorsion and fixation is the treatment of choice in order to afford the patient the highest chance of preserving gonadal function.

EPIDIDYMO-ORCHITIS

Epididymo-orchitis is an infectious, inflammatory condition of the epididymis and testis. The condition may involve the epididymis (epididymitis) or testis (orchitis) alone, or may occur in combination, known as epididymo-orchitis. The etiology of this condition is usually bacterial though viral causes of orchitis are known (classically mumps). In sexually active men less than the age of 40, *N. gonorrhea* and *Chlamydia* are the most common pathogens whereas in men over the age of 40, *E. coli* tends to be most common.

HISTORY: Patients with epididymo-orchitis will often report a gradual onset, constant pain in the involved testis. Some may also report symptoms of a urinary tract infection (dysuria, urgency and frequency). A history of purulent penile discharge should prompt one to consider *N. gonorrhea* as the causative agent.

PHYSICAL EXAM: The physical exam of a patient with epididymo-orchitis may reveal a tender, edematous testicle with an abnormal, horizontal lie. According to Prehn's test (which has shown to be unreliable and is mostly now of historical interest only), elevation of the affected testis will result in some relief of pain in epididymo-orchitis. If epididymitis alone is present, one may appreciate an enlarged, tender epididymis located at the superior, posterior pole of the testis.

WORK-UP: A urine analysis may help detect the presence of bacteria and leukocytes within the urinary tract. However, ultrasound is used most commonly in order to evaluate for inflammatory changes in the testis and/or epididymis.

TREATMENT: The treatment for epididymo-orchitis is usually determined by the patient's age and history of sexual activity. If the patient is <40 and is sexually active, treatment for sexually-transmitted infections (STIs) is provided (usually ceftriaxone 250mg IM x1 followed by doxycycline 100mg by mouth twice a day for 14 days). Alternatively, if the patient is >40 and/or has risk factors for UTIs, treatment against *E. coli* with an agent such as ciprofloxacin for 10-14 days is provided. A confirmatory urine culture should be sent in all cases.

PELVIC INFLAMMATORY DISEASE

HISTORY: Patients with pelvic inflammatory disease (PID) may report unilateral (or rarely bilateral) lower abdominal or pelvic pain with or without a fever. There will usually be a history of being sexually active or a prior history of an STI.

PHYSICAL EXAM: Patients with PID will classically exhibit cervical motion tenderness; however, there are many women who will only exhibit mild to moderate tenderness on the pelvic exam and therefore there must be a high index of suspicion for this diagnosis, especially given the consequences of infertility and chronic pelvic pain. In cases of a tubo-ovarian abscess, one may appreciate fullness and tenderness in the affected adenexa. *Trichomonas* may cause the cervix to be markedly erythematous ("strawberry" cervix) along with exuding a malodorous, frothy yellow-green discharge.

WORK-UP: The diagnosis of PID is usually made clinically and confirmed with PCR testing for *N. gonorrhea* and *Chlamydia*. Ultrasound or CT can be used to diagnose a tubo-ovarian abscess.

TREATMENT: PID is often diagnosed on presumptive clinical grounds and treatment is oftentimes given on an empirical basis. As resistance patterns vary by geographic location and evolve over time, it is best to consult the current CDC guidelines with respect to the preferred treatment strategy. In patients who are ill-appearing or febrile or who have a tubo-ovarian abscess, admission for IV antibiotics is usually indicated.

CHAPTER 5: FLANK PAIN

Pain in either flank may oftentimes represent severe, life-threatening pathology – that owing to the obtuse location – is often missed or misdiagnosed as resulting from another, more benign condition. Considering this, the "dangerous differential" for flank pain includes:

- Leakage of an abdominal aortic aneurysm
- Pyelonephritis
- Nephrolithiasis (kidney stone)
- Pulmonary embolism
- Epidural abscess

LEAKAGE OF AN ABDOMINAL AORTIC ANEURYSM (AAA)

HISTORY: Patients with a leaking abdominal aortic aneurysm (AAA) may report mid-abdominal pain, back pain or flank pain. Indeed, since the aorta is a retroperitoneal structure, leakage from an AAA more often presents as back or flank pain rather than abdominal pain. Patients may already carry a diagnosis of an AAA or may have risk factors for an AAA such as hypertension, hyperlipidemia, tobacco use and age greater than 50.

PHYSICAL EXAM: In patients with a lean body habitus, one may be able to appreciate a dilated abdominal aorta via deep abdominal palpation. While this will not indicate whether or not the aneurysm is leaking, a palpable aorta over 3cm in diameter will qualify as an AAA. In patients with a leaking AAA, the triad of hypotension, abdominal pain and a palpable pulsatile abdominal mass are sufficient to make a presumptive diagnosis.

WORK-UP: While most AAAs are discovered via ultrasound or CT of the abdomen/pelvis, the diagnosis of a ruptured or leaking AAA should be made upon clinical grounds. Occasionally, if the patient is somewhat stable, a CT abdomen/pelvis with IV contrast can help make the diagnosis of a leaking AAA.

TREATMENT: While asymptomatic AAAs >5.5cm can be referred to vascular surgery on an outpatient basis for open vs. endovascular repair, a leaking/ruptured AAA is an acute surgical emergency and the patient should go to the OR as soon as possible. Blood should be sent for type and crossmatch as soon as possible since the patient will likely require intraoperative blood transfusions.

PYELONEPHRITIS

HISTORY: Patients with pyelonephritis will usually report a gradual onset, constant pain in the flank without radiation, usually associated with a fever, headache, nausea/vomiting as well as dysuria, urgency and frequency. Patients tend to be female, though it is quite possible that you will encounter males with pyelonephritis especially if they are elderly, diabetic or have obstructive defects in their urinary tract.

PHYSICAL EXAM: Patients with pyelonephritis will often have a fever and will exhibit costo-vertebral angle tenderness on the affected site. Depending upon the severity of the infection, they may manifest signs and symptoms of sepsis.

WORK-UP: The diagnosis of pyelonephritis is largely clinical with a urine analysis offering supporting evidence of an infection somewhere along the urinary tract.

TREATMENT: The treatment of pyelonephritis is with antibiotics in addition to supportive measures such as hydration and fever reduction. Patients who are pregnant, diabetic, septic or unable to tolerate oral intake should be admitted for parenteral antibiotics.

NEPHROLITHIASIS (KIDNEY STONE)

While not particularly acutely life-threatening, nephrolithiasis causes such severe pain and occurs with enough frequency as to merit further consideration here.

HISTORY: Patients with nephrolithiasis often report an acute onset of severe pain in the flank that radiates to the ipsilateral groin. Nausea and vomiting are commonly associated. Hematuria is mostly microscopic, though some patients may report gross hematuria. Most patients with kidney stones that you will encounter will already carry a diagnosis of nephrolithiasis as this tends to be a recurring phenomenon.

PHYSICAL EXAM: Patients will tend to be in severe pain. The abdominal exam tends to be rather benign and any costo-vertebral angle tenderness will tend to be mild unless the patient has significant hydronephrosis from a large distal obstructing stone.

WORK-UP: In patients without a prior history of nephrolithiasis, CT of the abdomen/pelvis without contrast is the preferred method of diagnosis as it demonstrates the exact location of obstruction as well as indicates the size of the stone. However, for patients who already have an established history of nephrolithiasis and are presenting in a similar fashion, it is best to avoid CT in order to limit exposure to ionizing radiation. One may instead use ultrasound to evaluate for the presence of hydroureter and hydronephrosis (which would suggest a larger stone and therefore the need for more urgent urology follow-up). Ultrasound can be combined with a KUB x-ray to positively identify a radio-opaque stone. Urine analysis can help detect microscopic hematuria, but this is only approximately 60% sensitive for nephrolithiasis.

TREATMENT: Treatment of nephrolithiasis depends upon the size of the stone. Stones <4mm in diameter are managed conservatively with encouragement of good oral hydration and pain control, preferably with NSAIDs. Stones of larger size likely need to be referred to urology for further management such as endoscopic shock wave lithotripsy or nephrostomy tube placement. Agents such as tamsulosin or calcium channel blockers (medical expulsive therapy) have been shown in several trials to increase the passage rate of kidney stones[*].

---

[*] Singh A, et al. A systematic review of medical therapy to facilitate passage of ureteral calculi. *Ann Emerg Med.* 2007; 50(5): 552-63.

CHAPTER 6: BACK PAIN

You will surely encounter many patients whose chief complaint is back pain. While the vast majority of these will be suffering from musculoskeletal causes of their back pain, in the emergency department, our function is to identify those patients whose symptoms may be due to a more acute life- or limb-threatening source. When considering back pain, the "dangerous differential" should include:

- Cord compression
- Cauda equina syndrome
- Epidural abscess
- Vertebral osteomyelitis/discitis
- Malignancy
- Vertebral fracture
- Leaking or ruptured AAA

CORD COMPRESSION

HISTORY: Patients with compression of their spinal cord will often complain of back pain plus a loss of motor and/or sensory function distal to the level of compression. Oftentimes, they may report a "sensory level" – a clear line demarcating the point beyond which their sensation is diminished. Patients will most commonly experience compression of their cord from an overlying abscess (epidural abscess) or from a malignant tumor. Therefore, a relevant past medical history (such as IVDU or history of prostate cancer) may help make this diagnosis.

PHYSICAL EXAM: Patients may or may not exhibit tenderness in the midline at the point of compression depending upon the underlying etiology of the compression. However, a careful neurological exam may reveal a sensory level as well as motor deficits distal to the area of compression. Indeed, the presence of such neurological deficits should greatly increase one's suspicion of cord compression.

WORK-UP: Cord compression is typically diagnosed via MRI of the affected level of the spinal cord, which is in turn determined by the physical exam findings.

TREATMENT: Depending on the underlying reason for cord compression, treatment strategies can include radiation therapy to decrease the size of the compressing tumor versus surgery to either excise the impinging tumor or drain the epidural abscess.

CAUDA EQUINA SYNDROME

Cauda equina syndrome is similar in pathophysiology to cord compression and differs only in the location where compression is occurring. Namely, in cauda equina syndrome, the nerve roots of the lower lumbar and sacral regions are involved as the spinal cord itself terminates at a higher level (at the conus medullaris near L1/2).

HISTORY: Patients with cauda equina syndrome will first experience an inability to urinate and will eventually experience overflow incontinence. This is due to interruption of the sacral parasympathetic input that would ordinarily allow normal micturition. Eventually, with involvement of sufficient nerve roots, symptoms such as loss of perineal sensation and stool continence may occur.

PHYSICAL EXAM: One of the most sensitive indicators of cauda equina syndrome is an elevated post-void residual volume of urine. In addition, one may note the presence of a diminished or absent rectal tone as well as loss of sensation in the perineal distribution. Patients may or may not have midline lower back tenderness, depending upon the underlying etiology for the cauda equina syndrome.

WORK-UP: Once the diagnosis is suspected based on history and exam findings, MR is the preferred imaging modality to confirm the diagnosis.

TREATMENT: Treatment depends, once again, upon the underlying etiology of the cauda equina syndrome. However, neurosurgery should be consulted as soon as the diagnosis is suspected since time is of the essence in potentially preserving as much function as possible.

EPIDURAL ABSCESS

HISTORY: Patients suffering from an epidural abscess will usually report a high fever as well as mid back pain. If there is cord compression, they may additionally report various neurological symptoms such as sensory and motor deficits distal to the level of compression. Moreover, patients with an epidural abscess will likely demonstrate risk factors for the development of such an abscess such as IV drug abuse, alcoholism or immunocompromising conditions (diabetes, HIV).

PHYSICAL EXAM: The physical exam of a patient with an epidural abscess will likely reveal the presence of a fever along with marked tenderness in the mid-back. Patients will often experience pain that seems out of proportion to the rest of their history and exam. One should be diligent in searching for physical signs of risks factors for an epidural abscess such as track marks from IV drug abuse since such history might not be readily forthcoming from the patient.

WORK-UP: Once again, MR is the preferred imaging modality to diagnose an epidural abscess and can indicate the degree of cord impingement, if any.

TREATMENT: The treatment of an epidural abscess involves a combination of parenteral antibiotics and surgical drainage of the abscess.

VERTEBRAL OSTEOMYELITIS/DISCITIS

HISTORY: Patients with vertebral osteomyelitis usually have an indolent history of back pain that gradually increases with time. As with epidural abscess formation, the patient may exhibit risk factors for the development of vertebral osteomyelitis such as IV drug abuse, advanced age and immunocompromising conditions. Indeed, epidural abscess can be a complication of unchecked vertebral osteomyelitis. Seeding of bacteria is usually in the vertebral body rather than the posterior elements and tends to be hematogenous in origin.

PHYSICAL EXAM: Patients with vertebral osteomyelitis may exhibit only mild tenderness to palpation of the back, as it is the vertebral body that is most commonly involved rather that the more readily palpable posterior column elements. Fever is present in about one-half of patients and therefore is not a reliable discriminator of this disease process. If the osteomyelitis is advanced and collapse of the vertebral column elements occurs, symptoms of neurologic compromise may be evident on the exam.

WORK-UP: Patients with vertebral osteomyelitis may exhibit an elevated peripheral WBC count as well an elevated ESR/CRP. However, these features are relatively non-specific and MRI tends to be the diagnostic modality of choice when this condition is suspected.

TREATMENT: In most cases, vertebral osteomyelitis is treated with long-term broad-spectrum antibiotics, including coverage for MRSA as most cases of this disease are due to *S. aureus*. Surgical therapy might be required in cases refractory to medical management.

MALIGNANCY

HISTORY: Back pain due to malignancy is usually from a lesion metastatic to the spine rather than from a tumor primarily originating from spinal elements. Common cancer types that metastasize to the spine include prostate, breast, lung, renal and thyroid. Therefore, patients with these malignancies should be considered at especially high risk of having a malignant cause of their back pain.

PHYSICAL EXAM: The physical exam of a person with back pain due to a tumor will often reveal tenderness along the spine. They may also manifest signs indicative of the underlying malignancy (e.g. hemoptysis in the case of primary lung cancer).

WORK-UP: Metastatic lesions to the spine may cause an elevation in ESR. However, the diagnosis is often made on CT or MRI of the involved spine.

TREATMENT: Radiation therapy can be used to reduce the bulk of the tumor. Palliation of pain with an aggressive pain management protocol is also indicated.

CHAPTER 7: HEADACHE

Headache is one of the most commonly seen complaints among patients presenting to the emergency department. While most of these patients will have a primary headache syndrome (i.e. tension, migraine or cluster headache), it is the responsibility of the emergency department to ensure that the patient's headache is not secondary to a dangerous underlying condition. Some of these dangerous conditions include:

- Subarachnoid hemorrhage
- Meningitis
- Temporal arteritis
- Glaucoma
- Carbon monoxide toxicity
- Dural venous sinus thrombosis
- Tumor
- Subdural hematoma
- Epidural hematoma

SUBARACHNOID HEMORRHAGE

HISTORY: Patients with a spontaneous subarachnoid hemorrhage (SAH) will often relate a history of an acute, "thunderclap-onset" headache that was maximal at onset. Depending upon the extent of hemorrhage, patients may only complain of a headache or may experience seizures, alteration in mental status, syncope or complain of focal neurological deficits.

PHYSICAL EXAM: The physical exam for SAH may be rather benign if the hemorrhage is small. People with large hemorrhages or hemorrhages in sensitive locations may be found to have an alteration in consciousness and/or focal neurological findings.

WORK-UP: CT Head can pick up most hemorrhages if performed within 6 hours of headache onset. However, given the life-threatening nature of SAH, if the CT is negative, one must conduct a lumbar puncture (LP) to evaluate for the presence of blood or xanthochromia in order to rule-out subarachnoid hemorrhage with acceptable confidence. A CT Angiogram of the brain may also be done in order to discover possible culprit aneurysms.

TREATMENT: If a SAH is diagnosed and the patient is found to have a cerebral aneurysm or an arteriovenous malformation, surgical clipping or coiling may be undertaken to reduce the chance that a recurrent hemorrhage will occur.

MENINGITIS

HISTORY: Patients with meningitis will often report headache, fever, photophobia and nausea. With certain types of bacterial meningitis such as *N. meningitidis*, a history of living in close proximity to others (such as army barracks or college dorms) may be related. The patient may also report neck stiffness.

PHYSICAL EXAM: The patient with classic bacterial meningitis will exhibit nuchal rigidity with limitation of neck movement due to pain. Classic signs such as the Kernig and Brudzinski signs have been shown to be poorly reliable for meningitis. In contrast, the jolt accentuation test (having the patient rapidly turn their head from side to side and asking them if this makes their headache worse) has been shown to be rather sensitive, though poorly specific, for meningitis.

WORK-UP: Lumbar puncture and CSF analysis remain the mainstays of diagnosis. If this diagnosis is clinically suspected, antibiotics should be started immediately and not delayed until after the lumbar puncture. A gram stain, if positive, can give an early indication as to the causative organism.

TREATMENT: Most cases of bacterial meningitis are due to either *S. pneumoniae* or *N. meningitidis* with *H. influenzae* becoming much less prevalent after the introduction of the HIB vaccine. A typical antibiotic regimen would include ceftriaxone 2gm IV as well as vancomycin 1gm IV.

TEMPORAL ARTERITIS

HISTORY: This is predominantly a disease of those over the age of 50. Patients may report a throbbing temporal area headache. Since this headache is mediated by a medium-artery vasculitis (temporal arteritis is also known as giant cell arteritis), involvement of the ophthalmic artery may cause the patient to exhibit transient or even permanent blindness. Some patients may report associated muscle and joint aches (polymyalgia rheumatica)

PHYSICAL EXAM: The physical exam of a patient with temporal arteritis will reveal an oftentimes tender and pulseless temporal artery. If the ophthalmic artery is occluded, one may see a "cherry red spot" on the macula via direct ophthalmoscopy.

WORK-UP: An elevated ESR > 50-100 lends further evidence in support of this diagnosis. Definitive diagnosis is made by temporal artery biopsy, however treatment should be started on an empiric basis and not delayed until after the biopsy is performed.

TREATMENT: Treatment for temporal arteritis relies upon the use of high dose steroids. Patients may be discharged home on steroids until their biopsy can be performed as long as careful education about the use of steroids is provided to the patient (risks of hyperglycemia, sleep and psychiatric disturbances, premature cataracts and avascular necrosis, etc.) is provided.

GLAUCOMA (ACUTE ANGLE CLOSURE)

HISTORY: Patients with acute angle closure glaucoma often report the acute onset of a anterior or temporal headache. While some patients may be able to localize the symptoms to the eye, the intensity of the pain may lead other patients to believe that the pathology is intracranial, thus reporting a "headache". Patients will often note a change in their vision and classically acute angle closure glaucoma is precipitated by entry into a dark room which causes the pupil to dilate, blocking Schlemm's canal and thereby limiting aqueous humor outflow.

PHYSICAL EXAM: The physical exam of a patient with acute angle-closure glaucoma classically reveals a mid-size, non-reactive pupil with a "steamy-appearing" cornea. The affected eye will often feel more firm, or tense, than the contralateral eye.

WORK-UP: Tonometry will often reveal an elevated anterior chamber pressure. Readings of >20 mmHg are indicative of a higher than normal intraocular pressure.

TREATMENT: Treatment relies upon the use of pro-cholinergic drops such as pilocarpine, beta-blockers such as timolol and diuretics such as acetazolamide and mannitol. Anterior chamber paracentesis can also be performed in order to relieve pressure from the anterior chamber, but this procedure is best deferred to the ophthalmologist.

CARBON MONOXIDE TOXICITY

HISTORY: History is the key in making this diagnosis. Patients with CO-poisoning may not recognize their toxic exposure. Instead they may report vague complaints of headache, nausea and flu-like symptoms of acute onset. Multiple family members presenting with the same vague symptoms is oftentimes a clue to CO-poisoning.

PHYSICAL EXAM: The physical exam of a patient with CO-poisoning can be rather benign. Patients will sometimes exhibit "cherry-red" lips due to failure of oxygen to uncouple from hemoglobin leading to a falsely high pulse oximetry reading.

WORK-UP: The diagnosis is often made on the basis of history, however an arterial blood gas with co-oximetry can confirm the diagnosis by demonstrating an elevated carboxyhemoglobin level.

TREATMENT: In mild cases of CO-poisoning, the patient can be treated supportively with 100% O_2 delivered by non-rebreather mask. In cases of pregnancy, underlying pulmonary disease or severe poisoning with neurological effects, the patient should be placed in a hyperbaric oxygen chamber in order to displace CO from hemoglobin.

DURAL VENOUS SINUS THROMBOSIS

Dural venous sinus thrombosis involves a blood clot within the venous dural sinuses that drain deoxygenated blood from the brain. In certain instances, such as with cavernous sinus thrombosis, the thrombosis is due to an infectious source and the patient may manifest a fever along with neurological findings from pressure exerted by the thrombosis.

HISTORY: Patients with dural venous sinus thrombosis will often have hypercoagulability risk factors such as Factor V Leiden, Protein C or S deficiency, or Prothrombin G20210A mutation. If the thrombosis is from an infectious source such as in cavernous sinus thrombosis, the patient may have an infection of the midface such as facial cellulitis or sinusitis. Patients will often report a gradual onset, worsening headache often with focal neurological findings.

PHYSICAL EXAM: Depending on the location of the dural venous sinus thrombosis, the patient may exhibit focal neurological findings and/or exhibit a seizure. In cases of cavernous sinus thrombosis for instance, patients may have a fever, bilateral proptosis and/or abducens nerve palsy. As the disease progresses, other structures within the cavernous sinus may become involved such as the ophthalmic nerve (leading to a dilated and poorly reactive pupil), oculomotor nerve, trochlear nerve, and ophthalmic and maxillary branches of the fifth cranial nerve.

WORK-UP: Diagnosis is usually made by CT or MR venography which may demonstrate a thrombus within the affected dural venous sinus.

TREATMENT: In cases of an infectious thrombosis, IV antibiotics are rapidly administered. For non-infectious cases, anticoagulants such as heparin and warfarin can be administered.

TUMOR

HISTORY: An intracranial tumor is a rare but important cause of headache. Typically patients with an intracranial tumor will describe headaches that are worse in the morning and improve with sitting or standing up. Depending upon the size and location of the tumor, patients may report focal neurological symptoms and/or seizures.

PHYSICAL EXAM: The physical exam of a patient with an intracranial tumor varies depending upon the location and size of the tumor. Oftentimes, the patient will not have any noticeable focal neurological deficit on exam and the diagnosis will have to be suspected entirely on historical grounds. In more advanced cases, patients may demonstrate seizures, focal neurological deficits and/or an alteration in their normal pattern of behavior or consciousness.

WORK-UP: Tumors are often discovered by CT. Non-contrast CT can demonstrate a mass effect if the tumor is large enough. However, for tumors too small to cause a shift of surrounding structures, IV contrast is needed in order to detect the tumor. MR is the preferred diagnostic modality to confirm and further characterize an intracranial tumor.

TREATMENT: Treatment strategies vary depending upon the type, size and location of the tumor and a detailed consideration of treatments is beyond the scope of this writing.

SUBDURAL HEMORRHAGE

HISTORY: Subdural hemorrhage usually results from tearing of the bridging dural veins, resulting in blood collecting deep to the dura mater. Patients tend to be elderly, on anticoagulants and may relate a history of a recent fall. It is important to note that sometimes subdural hemorrhages evolve over a period of hours to days therefore a headache may not develop until a significant period of time has elapsed after a fall.

PHYSICAL EXAM: The patient with a subdural hemorrhage may demonstrate focal neurological deficits and may be altered or may be surprisingly asymptomatic with no obvious physical exam findings.

WORK-UP: Subdural hemorrhage is classically identified by non-contrast CT demonstrating a concave, lenticular-shaped, extra-axial area of increased attenuation.

TREATMENT: Depending upon the patient's symptoms, management can range from simple observation to surgical drainage of the subdural blood.

EPIDURAL HEMORRHAGE

HISTORY: Patients with an epidural hemorrhage will classically relate a history of significant temporo-parietal head trauma immediately followed by a loss of consciousness with a return to a "lucid interval" before experiencing a second, more profound loss of consciousness. The degree of trauma is usually much more severe in cases of epidural hemorrhage versus cases of subdural hemorrhage.

PHYSICAL EXAM: The physical exam of a patient with an epidural hemorrhage may reveal a fracture of the temporal skull as the pathophysiology of epidural hemorrhage involves disruption of the middle meningeal artery which runs along the inner table of the temporal portion of the cranium.

WORK-UP: The diagnosis of epidural hemorrhage is most commonly made by non-contrast CT imaging which reveals a convex shaped extradural area of increased attenuation representing blood collected in the epidural space, limited by the dural attachments. Epidural hemorrhages are commonly associated with skull fractures, especially of the temporal bone.

TREATMENT: Treatment of an epidural hemorrhage involves surgical evacuation of the epidural blood especially if early signs of uncal herniation are present on exam.

CHAPTER 8: ALTERED MENTAL STATUS

The evaluation of an alteration in mental status, or consciousness, can be quite complex. Consciousness can be thought of as being composed of two components: arousal and cognition. Arousal is dependent upon the ascending reticular activating system (ARAS) which is physically located in the midbrain. In contrast, cognition (memory, higher-level thought processes) relies upon the successful functioning of both cerebral hemispheres. Therefore, conditions affecting the ARAS often lead to coma whereas pathologies of the cerebral hemispheres often lead to focal neurological deficits and/or confusion. The imperative of the emergency department is to rapidly determine life-threatening causes of an alteration in mental status and to promptly institute corrective therapies. With this imperative in mind, the "dangerous differential" of a patient with altered mental status should include:

- Hypoglycemia
- Hypoxia
- Intoxication/withdrawal syndromes
- Wernicke's encephalopathy
- Intracranial hemorrhage
- Sepsis
- Electrolyte disturbances
- Thyroid emergencies
- Adrenal crisis
- Tumor

HYPOGLYCEMIA

HISTORY: Patients with hypoglycemia may carry a diagnosis of diabetes. As these patients are oftentimes altered, they will not be able to provide a salient history and one can look for the presence of medical bracelets which may carry such information. However, hypoglycemia occurs with such frequency that it should be entertained in the immediate differential of anyone presenting with an altered mental status.

PHYSICAL EXAM: Patients with hypoglycemia can have a myriad of clinical presentations. Classically, they will report palpitations, lightheadedness and diaphoresis. Patients may manifest a variety of focal neurological findings and may even act in a seemingly psychotic fashion. Therefore, the physical exam of a patient with hypoglycemia tends to be rather non-specific.

WORK-UP: The diagnosis can be rapidly ascertained by performing a bedside random blood glucose test.

TREATMENT: Patients with hypoglycemia should immediately be given glucose, preferably via IV (1 amp or 25mg) or by mouth if the patient is able to tolerate this. In patients in whom IV access is difficult, one may give 1mg of glucagon intramuscularly. Glucagon will increase glycogenolysis and gluconeogenesis from the liver. However, glucagon will be of limited efficacy in patients with hepatic cirrhosis.

HYPOXIA

HISTORY: Patients or family members may relate a history of previous pulmonary disease or may endorse experiencing a sudden airway obstruction. In most instances, patients will not be cognizant enough to provide a reliable history.

PHYSICAL EXAM: Patients with hypoxia will tend to be agitated and restless. They may manifest peripheral cyanosis. In contrast, patients with hypercarbia will often be somnolent and difficult to arouse.

WORK-UP: Pulse oximetry can rapidly indicate the patient's oxygen saturation. One must be careful of conditions such as carbon monoxide poisoning which can yield a falsely high pulse oximeter reading however. An arterial blood gas may be more useful in these cases. Once the patient is acutely stabilized, the work-up should focus on determining the underlying etiology of the hypoxia.

TREATMENT: Oxygen can be administered non-invasively by nasal cannula, face mask, non-rebreather mask or by continuous or bi-level positive airway pressure devices. If the patient's oxygenation does not improve with these methods, s/he may need to be intubated.

INTOXICATION/WITHDRAWAL SYNDROMES

There are literally hundreds of substances which can induce an alteration in mental status. Some of these have clearly definable toxidromes such as alcohol, opiates, anticholinergic, and pro-sympathetic agents, whereas poisoning by other agents may not be as clear without a reliable history. Withdrawal from substances such as alcohol, benzodiazepines and cocaine can also present with an alteration of consciousness among other features. For our introductory purposes, I will limit the ensuing discussion to alcohol and opiates since these are toxidromes that we are likely to repeatedly encounter.

HISTORY: Patients may or may not be forthcoming with a history or alcohol or opiate use, especially if they are experiencing an alteration in mental status. Again, one must rely upon information provided by collateral sources such as family members, paramedics and a patient's personal belongings (i.e. drug paraphernalia) to assist in elucidating an underlying etiology for the altered mental status.

PHYSICAL EXAM: The physical exam is perhaps the most important component of determining a potential toxidrome. Patients with opiate intoxication will often manifest bradypnea, meiosis and lethargy. Conversely, patients with alcohol intoxication may be inappropriately vasodilated, may exude an odor of liquor/beer and may exhibit signs of hepatic cirrhosis. Most importantly, one must examine the head and neck of such patients to evaluate for the presence of possible head trauma.

WORK-UP: While a urine toxicology screen or blood alcohol level can help confirm a diagnosis, the mainstay of diagnosis is still clinical as toxicology screens can remain positive weeks after last use and patients who are intoxicated may be altered due to an intracranial hemorrhage sustained during a fall while intoxicated.

TREATMENT: In patients with undifferentiated altered mental status, there is little harm in administering 0.2 to 0.4 mg of naloxone to assess for a response. If a patient returns to baseline, a diagnosis of opiate intoxication is very likely. For patients with alcohol intoxication, only supportive measures are routinely indicated. Vitamin supplementation can be considered since many of these patients are nutritionally poor.

WERNICKE'S ENCEPHALOPATHY

HISTORY: Patients with Wernicke's encephalopathy will often have a history of long-standing alcoholism. However, due to the psychosis common with this disorder as well as due to the confusion and amnesia associated with Korsakoff syndrome, histories from these patients may not be reliable.

PHYSICAL EXAM: The classic triad of Wernicke's syndrome consists of ataxia, psychosis and ophthalmoplegia (paralysis of eye movements). Korsakoff syndrome is thought to be on the irreversible end of the spectrum of Wernicke-Korsakoff syndrome with confabulation and amnesia as predominant symptoms.

WORK-UP: The Wernicke-Korsakoff syndrome is thought to be due to a deficiency of thiamine (vitamin B1). While levels of thiamine can be checked, from the emergency department standpoint, the diagnosis should be made clinically and treatment started empirically.

TREATMENT: Patients suspected of having Wernicke's encephalopathy should receive 100mg of IV Thiamine. The previous admonition to administer thiamine only *after* glucose has been given has not been shown to be necessary. Therefore, thiamine should be administered as soon as the diagnosis is considered or alternatively, can be administered to everyone with undifferentiated altered mental status as a part of the "coma cocktail": Dextrose, Oxygen, Naloxone, Thiamine.

INTRACRANIAL HEMORRHAGE

HISTORY: Patients with an intracranial hemorrhage as the source of their altered mental status may report a history of recent head trauma or may be able to relate that they had an acute onset severe headache.

PHYSICAL EXAM: One should be diligent in searching for clues of head trauma in patients with altered mental status. The skull should be palpated for any step-offs and to detect any blood from an occult scalp laceration. Classic signs of a basilar skull fracture include periorbital ecchymosis (raccoon eyes), ecchymosis over the mastoid process (Battle sign), hemotympanum and CSF oto- or rhinorrhea.

WORK-UP: A CT of the head may detect the presence of an intracranial hemorrhage. In cases of a suspected spontaneous SAH, a negative CT does not have enough sensitivity to rule-out the diagnosis and a lumbar puncture evaluating for the presence of blood or xanthochromia within the CSF should be performed.

TREATMENT: Treatment can range from simple observation, administration of anticoagulation reversal agents to surgical evacuation of intracranial blood depending upon the patient's particular symptoms.

ELECTROLYTE DISTURBANCES

Electrolyte disturbances such as hypo- and hypernatremia and hypercalcemia are frequent causes of altered mental status, especially among the elderly. These metabolic causes of an altered mental status tend to cause more diffuse neurological symptoms (such as lethargy and confusion) rather than focal neurological findings.

HISTORY: Family members may relate a history of poor water intake or the patient may be taking diuretic medications which can precipitate hyponatremia. The patient may also have a known underlying malignancy which could be the cause of hypercalcemia and may report other associated symptoms such as diffuse abdominal pain and a history of kidney stones.

PHYSICAL EXAM: The physical exam can offer clues as to the presence of an underlying electrolyte disturbance. For instance, in severe hyponatremia, the skin may take on a rather "doughy" consistency whereas in hypercalcemia the patient may exhibit hyperreflexia and fasciculation of the tongue.

WORK-UP: The diagnosis of these conditions relies upon obtaining a serum electrolyte panel.

TREATMENT: Hyponatremia can be treated with water restriction in most cases, though hypertonic saline may be given in cases of seizures or an acute change in mental status. Hypernatremia is treated by free water replacement. Hypercalcemia is initially treated by giving IV fluids and non-thiazide diuretics to dilute, and then remove, the excess calcium. Bisphosphonates and steroids are also often given in the treatment of hypercalcemia.

THYROID EMERGENCIES

Hyper- and hypothyroidism in their extreme states, thyrotoxicosis and myxedema coma, respectively, can both lead to an alteration in mental status. Typically thyrotoxic patients will be agitated whereas patients with myxedema may be rather lethargic.

HISTORY: Patients or family members may report a past medical history of thyroid disease or a review of medications can help suggest the diagnosis if the patient or family are unable to provide much information. Particular attention should be given to pre-existing symptoms of hyper- or hypothyroidism, as a diagnosis may not have yet been made.

PHYSICAL EXAM: Patients with hyperthyroidism may exhibit proptosis, atrial fibrillation, diaphoresis, tachycardia, tachypnea and an elevated core temperature. Conversely, patients with myxedema may demonstrate brawny, non-pitting lower extremity edema, a delayed relaxation phase with respect to their deep tendon reflexes, bradycardia and hypotension. Oftentimes, there is an underlying infection that acts as a precipitant of the thyroid storm or myxedema coma and signs of such an infection should be sought on the exam.

WORK-UP: The diagnosis must typically be made upon clinical grounds as treatment often cannot be delayed until the results of detailed laboratory testing are available. However, a TSH and free T4 level can help confirm the diagnosis once it returns.

TREATMENT: Treatment firstly focuses on the underlying cause of the thyroid storm or myxedema coma (i.e. antibiotics for the precipitating infection). Thyrotoxicosis is treated with a combination of propranolol, propylthiouracil (PTU), iodine (only after PTU is given) and dexamethasone. Treatment for myxedema coma relies upon the IV replacement of thyroxine.

ADRENAL CRISIS

HISTORY: Patients with adrenal crisis will often be on long-standing steroids or will have recently completed a long-term steroid taper (usually longer than 10-14 days). As an infectious etiology usually precipitates the crisis, patients may report symptoms of an infection (such as cough, fever, etc.).

PHYSICAL EXAM: Patients experiencing an adrenal crisis will often appear to be rather ill. Nausea and vomiting are frequent symptoms. Patients will tend to be hypotensive and tachycardic while being inappropriately vasodilated. These signs may mimic a septic state.

WORK-UP: A history of being on recent long-term steroids is invaluable in making the diagnosis. Laboratory results will often indicate hyponatremia, hyperkalemia, acidosis and hypoglycemia. A random cortisol level can be drawn and will oftentimes be low.

TREATMENT: Providing both mineralocorticoid and glucocorticoid replacement is essential. Therefore steroids such as methylprednisolone are ideal. In patients without much electrolyte disturbance, a pure glucocorticoid such as dexamethasone may suffice.

TUMOR

HISTORY: As indicated in the section on headaches, patients with altered mental status as a result of a CNS neoplasm will often report headaches that are worse in the mornings and which improve with standing up. The headache will tend to be of several weeks or months in duration and family members may note the presence of subtle personality changes.

PHYSICAL EXAM: Since a neoplastic process is a structural abnormality within the CNS, one may expect to find focal neurological findings on a careful exam. If there is obstruction by the neoplasm of the ventricular system, papilledema may be appreciated on direct ophthalmoscopy. If the neoplasm is metastatic to the CNS from another source, physical findings consistent with the primary neoplastic process may be encountered (i.e. melanoma skin lesion).

WORK-UP: CT with contrast and/or MRI can be used to diagnose intracranial masses. Non-contrast CT may demonstrate a mass if it is large enough to cause a shift in the normal anatomical location of adjacent structures (i.e. mass effect).

TREATMENT: Treatment depends upon the exact tumor type, location and attributable symptoms.

CHAPTER 9: SORE THROAT

While a common and seemingly benign chief complaint, there are several "dangerous" pathologies to consider in patients presenting to the emergency department with a chief complaint of sore throat:

- Peritonsillar abscess
- Deep space neck infections (para-, retropharyngeal, prevertebral neck abscesses)
- Ludwig's angina
- Epiglottitis
- Diphtheria
- Candidiasis
- Lemierre's syndrome

PERITONSILLAR ABSCESS

HISTORY: Patients with a peritonsillar cellulitis or abscess will usually report a unilateral sore throat with fever along with odynophagia (painful swallowing). Patients may have a past history of Group A β-hemolytic streptococcal (GABHS) pharyngitis.

PHYSICAL EXAM: The physical exam will reveal medial and inferior displacement of the affected tonsil along with fullness in the peritonsillar space representing the location of the abscess. One may also note submandibular and cervical lymphadenopathy along with possible exudates on the tonsil. The patient's voice may be muffled.

WORK-UP: The diagnosis is predominantly clinical though CT imaging with IV contrast can help distinguish between an abscess and cellulitis and can demonstrate the extent of the abscess, if any.

TREATMENT: Peritonsillar abscesses are treated by drainage in the emergency department. Care must be taken to incise the abscess along its medial border as the carotid artery and internal jugular vein are just lateral and deep to the peritonsillar space. Antibiotics covering GABHS and *S. aureus* are indicated as well. Patients unable to tolerate oral intake should be admitted for IV antibiotics. Patients are typically referred to ENT on an outpatient basis for consideration for further drainage and eventual tonsillectomy.

DEEP SPACE NECK INFECTIONS

This group of disorders includes peritonsillar abscess (discussed above), parapharyngeal abscess, retropharyngeal abscess and pre-vertebral space abscess. Abscesses in these locations tend to be dangerous in that they may occlude the airway and may provide a direct path for bacteria into the mediastinum. Organisms responsible are typically streptococcal and staphylococcal species and antibiotic choice should reflect this prevalence.

HISTORY: Patients with a deep space neck infection may report a progressively worsening sore throat along with fevers. Patients with para-, retropharyngeal and prevertebral space infections may also demonstrate neck stiffness owing to the proximity of these abscesses to the cervical muscles. As with peritonsillar abscesses, patients may report odynophagia and may have difficulty tolerating their secretions.

PHYSICAL EXAM: Due to the raphe formed by the superior constrictor muscle, retropharyngeal abscesses tend to be off the midline while pre-vertebral space abscesses will be in the midline. Parapharyngeal abscesses are adjacent to the carotid sheath and may cause fullness in the area of the carotid and posterior triangles.

WORK-UP: The above deep space neck infections are usually diagnosed by CT with intravenous contrast. However, if a patient is in acute respiratory distress, airway control should be secured before obtaining a CT.

TREATMENT: As with most abscesses, treatment involves incision and drainage of the offending abscess. IV antibiotics covering streptococcal and staphylococcal species should be promptly initiated. In patients with respiratory distress and impending airway occlusion, airway control must be established as quickly and as safely as possible. Preferably, these patients should be intubated in the operating room using fiberoptic laryngoscopy with tools for a surgical airway (cricothyrotomy or tracheostomy) at the ready.

LUDWIG'S ANGINA

Lugwig's angina is a cellulitis of the soft tissues located in the submandibular, sublingual and submental spaces. The resultant edema and induration of tissues elevates the tongue and displaces it posteriorly, potentially causing it to occlude the airway.

HISTORY: Patients with Ludwig's angina typically will report a history of a recent mandibular dental infection. Indeed, most causes of Ludwig's angina start off as a mandibular dental infection that breaks through the mandibular cortex and spreads along facial planes in the submandibular space. Patients may demonstrate a "hot potato" voice and may report trouble tolerating secretions.

PHYSICAL EXAM: Patients with Ludwig's angina may demonstrate a "bull neck" due to edema and induration of submandibular space soft tissues. The tongue will appear enlarged and elevated on oral examination. One may also note the presence of a foul odor emanating from the mouth and if anaerobic, gas-forming species are involved, crepitus may be noted. Patients may also exhibit a fever. In general, there will only be induration without fluctuance as Lugwig's angina is predominantly a *cellulitis* of the submandibular tissues rather than a frank abscess.

WORK-UP: The diagnosis should be made on clinical grounds, though contrast-enhanced CT will also demonstrate fullness in the submandibular space.

TREATMENT: Prompt airway control is paramount as most cases of death in Ludwig's angina occur from asphyxiation secondary to airway occlusion by the tongue. Therefore airway control should be approached with fiberoptic intubation and if unsuccessful or unavailable, a surgical airway should be performed (cricothyrotomy or tracheostomy). IV antibiotics covering streptococcal and staphylococcal species along with anaerobic coverage should be provided. Regimens such as high dose IV penicillin G with metronidazole or clindamycin should suffice.

Epiglottitis

HISTORY: While epiglottitis is classically a disease of childhood, the incidence has dropped considerably after the advent of the HIB vaccine. Therefore, relatively more adults are being diagnosed with this condition than children. Patients may report several days of throat pain along with a fever. In most severe cases, patients may report dyspnea, odynophagia and trouble swallowing their secretions. Oftentimes, sore throat is the only complaint elaborated by the patient.

PHYSICAL EXAM: The routine oral exam of a patient with epiglottis may be rather benign. However, the patient will report symptoms out of proportion with these exam findings. Oftentimes, there is pain with manipulation of the larynx. Fiberoptic laryngoscopy may reveal inflammation of the epiglottis and/or supraglottic tissues.

WORK-UP: While plain lateral neck radiographs may demonstrate edema of the epiglottis, the only reliable way to diagnose this condition is via laryngoscopy. CT can also demonstrate edema of the supraglottic tissues, but one must be careful not to send patients with a potentially unstable airway out of the emergency department for a diagnostic study.

TREATMENT: As with most infections of the neck, airway control is paramount. Intubation can be performed via direct laryngoscopy, but preparation should be made for an emergent surgical airway. Most cases of epiglottitis are due to *H. influenzae* type B and agents such as cefotaxime and ceftriaxone will provide adequate coverage.

DIPHTHERIA

HISTORY: Patients with diphtheria pharyngitis will report having a severe sore throat and may also report a descending muscular weakness as well as possible chest pain due to the predilection of diphtheria to cause myocarditis. Since *C. diphtheriae* is spread via person-to-person contact, patients may report contact with an infected individual.

PHYSICAL EXAM: Patients with pharyngeal diphtheria will usually exhibit a greyish membrane coating the posterior pharynx composed of neutrophils, fibrin, erythrocytes and bacteria. It is this pseudomembrane that is responsible for death via asphyxiation in diphtheria. In addition, one may note the presence of muscular weakness since an exotoxin elaborated by the bacterium causes neurotoxicity. In addition, an irregular cardiac rhythm may be appreciated due to diphtheric myocarditis.

WORK-UP: Definitive diagnosis is made by culture on Löffler's or tellurite media. However, a presumptive diagnosis should be made on clinical grounds and treatment initiated.

TREATMENT: The mainstay of treatment for diphtheria is with diphtheria antitoxin as well as macrolide antibiotics. The airway should be secured if there is any question of potential compromise from the inflammatory/exudative process.

CANDIDIASIS

HISTORY: Patients with oropharyngeal candidiasis may report a past history of an immunocompromising condition such as HIV or recent chemotherapy. They may report odynophagia and may have noted the presence of white patches on their pharynx.

PHYSICAL EXAM: Oropharynygeal candidiasis will likely result in an erythematous pharynx often with white plaques that are easily removed by light blunt debridement. If there is esophageal involvement, the patient may note retrosternal pain upon swallowing.

WORK-UP: The diagnosis tends to be clinical though fungal culture or visualization of removed plaques under light microscopy can be used to confirm the diagnosis.

TREATMENT: Treatment can be accomplished with oral fluconazole or with topical antifungals such as nystatin. More importantly, efforts should be directed at identifying and possibly reversing the underlying immunocompromising condition.

LEMIERRE'S SYNDROME

Lemierre's syndrome results from a septic thrombophlebitis of the internal jugular vein with resultant septic emboli, principally to the lungs, but potentially also throughout the systemic circulation. The cause is thought to be due to a pharyngitis caused by the bacterium *Fusobacterium necrophorum* that subsequently spreads to the parapharyngeal space and later causes septic thrombophlebitis of the internal jugular vein.

HISTORY: Patients with Lemierre's syndrome often report a recent history of having a non-specific pharyngitis. By the time of presentation, patients tend to be quite ill-appearing and may report cough (from septic pulmonary emboli) as well as joint pains, a vesiculopustular rash, CNS symptoms and soft tissue abscesses resulting from systemic septic emboli.

PHYSICAL EXAM: Patients with this syndrome will tend to be febrile and rather ill-appearing. Tenderness may be elicited with palpable along the carotid sheath on the affected side. In addition, the patient may have bilateral pulmonary crackles as well as evidence of systemic septic emboli. The clinical presentation may mimic that of bacterial endocarditis, however the source of the septic emboli in Lemierre's syndrome is from an infected internal jugular vein rather than primary cardiac valvular vegetations.

WORK-UP: The diagnosis of Lemierre's syndrome is often challenging since it tends to mimic bacterial endocarditis. However a history of a recent pharyngitis as well as tenderness along the carotid sheath may help clinch the diagnosis.

TREATMENT: Broad-spectrum antibiotics, including anaerobic coverage, should be administered until a causative organism is isolated from blood cultures. In patients who continue to experience septic emboli despite aggressive parenteral antibiotics, the affected internal jugular vein may need to be ligated and resected to eliminate the source of infection.

CHAPTER 10: EXTREMITY PAIN

Patients can experience pain in an extremity from a myriad of causes. More commonly, these are related to trauma (fracture, contusion) or overuse (muscular strain/sprain). However, there are many causes of non-traumatic extremity pain that need to be promptly diagnosed and intervened upon in order to mitigate a loss of function. Some such conditions representing a "dangerous differential" of pain in an extremity are:

- Deep venous thrombosis
- Necrotizing fasciitis
- Compartment syndrome
- Acute arterial insufficiency
- Septic arthritis

DEEP VENOUS THROMBOSIS

HISTORY: Patients with a deep venous thrombosis (DVT) of their extremity will likely report a history of prolonged immobilization followed by swelling and pain in the affected extremity. Some patients with inherited thrombophilias may report a positive family or personal history of previous DVTs and possible pulmonary emboli.

PHYSICAL EXAM: The physical exam of a patient with a lower extremity DVT may reveal asymmetric edema along with palpable and tender venous cords. Classic tests such as Homan's sign (pain in the calf with dorsiflexion of the foot) have been shown to be unreliable.

WORK-UP: The Wells Criteria are used to establish a pre-test probability for DVT. Patients with a low-risk Wells score should undergo d-dimer testing. Those patients with a high-risk Wells score or positive d-dimer should then undergo duplex ultrasonography.

TREATMENT: DVTs can be treated on an outpatient basis with enoxaparin if the patient is otherwise stable and able to comply with treatment. Patients are then bridged to treatment with warfarin to reduce the risk of DVT recurrence.

NECROTIZING FASCIITIS

HISTORY: Patients with necrotizing fasciitis usually have a history of an immunocompromising condition such as diabetes, chronic alcoholism, etc. that predisposes them to this particularly aggressive infection. Patients may recall minor trauma to the skin before onset of the necrotizing infection. Patients will often report pain that is out of proportion to exam findings.

PHYSICAL EXAM: Patients with necrotizing fasciitis may exhibit pain out of proportion to exam, lymphangitic streaking, hemorrhagic bullae, crepitus, and areas of erythema "skipping" up the involved extremity. It is important to note that most patients will not manifest all or even most of these signs. Therefore, whenever a patient appears to have cellulitis, one must consider necrotizing fasciitis and look for corroborating evidence.

WORK-UP: The diagnosis of necrotizing fasciitis is of necessity clinical and surgical. If the diagnosis is being entertained, the patient should be taken to the operating room and an incision made to evaluate for the presence of necrosis along fascial planes. Hyponatremia is a commonly sited finding in necrotizing fasciitis but it is important to note that it is neither sensitive nor specific. CT of the extremity may demonstrate the presence of gas and may reveal the true extent of infection, but CT should not be routinely used to make this diagnosis as time is of the essence.

TREATMENT: Treatment of necrotizing fasciitis is predominantly surgical. However, broad-spectrum antibiotics with efficacy versus streptococcal and staphylococcal species as well as anaerobes should be initiated immediately. A regimen of piperacillin/tazobactam, vancomycin and clindamycin should be administered. In addition, the patient should be aggressively resuscitated. Therapies such as intravenous immunoglobin (IVIG) and hyperbaric oxygen remain controversial.

COMPARTMENT SYNDROME

Compartment syndrome occurs when the pressure within a fascial compartment exceeds the mean arterial pressure of the artery or arteries supplying that compartment and distal structures. Intra-compartmental pressures typically rise due to edema or hematoma formation from injury to tissues lying within that compartment.

HISTORY: Most patients suffering from compartment syndrome will relate a recent history of trauma to the involved extremity. They may report distal paresthesias, one of the earliest symptoms of compartment syndrome. As the pressure rises and arterial supply is reduced distally, the patient may report ischemic pain and loss of sensation and motor function distal to the affected compartment.

PHYSICAL EXAM: Patients with acute compartment syndrome early in the course may exhibit only pain with passive stretch of the compartment. However, as the disease progresses, one may note a temperature difference between the extremities along with diminished sensation and motor function. Lack of a distal pulse is a late finding in compartment syndrome. Typically the compartment will feel firm, though with the deep posterior compartment of the leg, due to its deep location, one may not appreciate a frank firmness upon palpation of the calf.

WORK-UP: Once the diagnosis is suspected upon clinical grounds, it is confirmed by measuring the intra-compartmental pressure with a special manometry device. Though the exact pressure indicating the presence of compartment syndrome is controversial, many sources use a pressure of 30 mmHg or a difference between the diastolic blood pressure and intra-compartmental pressure of ≤20 mmHg to indicate the presence of compartment syndrome.

TREATMENT: The treatment for acute compartment syndrome involves performing a fasciotomy in order to relieve the pressure within the relevant compartment.

ACUTE ARTERIAL INSUFFICIENCY

HISTORY: Patients with acute arterial insufficiency of a limb will usually complain of an acute onset of pain in the affected limb without preceding trauma. Oftentimes, these patients will have a source for the occluding embolus such as from atrial fibrillation or from an abdominal aortic aneurysm (AAA).

PHYSICAL EXAM: Patients with an acute arterial embolus to an extremity will often present with a cool, pulseless limb with decreased sensation. Patients will tend to be in significant pain from lactic acid build-up as a consequence of ischemia. If several hours have passed since the occlusion occurred, early necrosis of the distal limb may be apparent.

WORK-UP: The absence of pulses can be confirmed via Doppler ultrasound. Ultrasound may also help elucidate the location of the offending clot. More importantly, a search for the underlying cause of the embolus should be initiated so as to mitigate the risk of future emboli.

TREATMENT: The patient should promptly be started on heparin and vascular surgery consulted for either emergent revascularization or endovascular embolectomy.

SEPTIC ARTHRITIS

HISTORY: Patients with septic arthritis will often report severe pain in the affected joint such that they are no longer able to range the joint. Patients may also report fever. Some patients may carry a history that predisposes them to developing septic arthritis such as sickle cell anemia and IV drug abuse.

PHYSICAL EXAM: The physical exam of a patient with a true bacterial septic arthritis will reveal an irritable joint that is nearly impossible to range, even passively. The knee joint will demonstrate an effusion, will oftentimes be warm with overlying erythema and will demonstrate pain with axial loading. Patients with a history of IV drug abuse may manifest track marks while those with endocarditis as a source will likely exhibit a cardiac murmur.

WORK-UP: The diagnosis of a septic joint can be made by performing an arthrocetesis and sending the fluid obtained for cell count with differential, gram stain, culture and crystal analysis. While many non-infectious inflammatory arthropathies can cause an elevated synovial WBC, these non-infectious diseases (gout, pseudogout) will often demonstrate crystals and will have a negative gram stain and culture. It is important to note that even in cases of true bacterial septic arthritis the gram stain can be falsely negative and if there is any doubt, one should presume a bacterial infection until proven otherwise.

TREATMENT: The treatment for septic arthritis involves administration of parenteral antibiotics with orthopedic consultation for surgical irrigation of the affected joint. As the causative organisms tend to be staphylococci, streptococci, *N. meningitidis* or gram negative rods, a combination of ceftriaxone and vancomycin should suffice. In patients with sickle cell anemia who are predisposed to getting septic arthritis due to salmonella (though *S. aureus* is still more common), treatment with ciprofloxacin and vancomycin is warranted.

REFERENCES

Marx JA, Hockberger RS, Walls RM (eds): *Rosen's emergency medicine: concepts and clinical practice*, 6th ed., Philadelphia, 2006, Mosby.

Tintinalli JE, Kelen GD, Stapczynski JS (eds): *Emergency medicine: a comprehensive study guide*, 6th ed., New York, 2004, McGraw-Hill.

Wolfson AB, Hendey GW, Hendry PL, et al. (eds): *Harwood-Nuss' clinical practice of emergency medicine*, 4th ed., Philadelphia, 2006, Lippincott Williams & Wilkins.

www.ingramcontent.com/pod-product-compliance
Lightning Source LLC
Chambersburg PA
CBHW081305170526
45165CB00011B/3422